CHINESE HERBAL MEDICINE

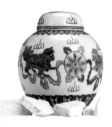

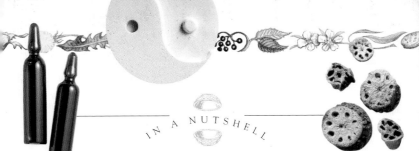

IN A NUTSHELL

CHINESE
HERBAL MEDICINE
A STEP-BY-STEP
GUIDE

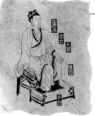

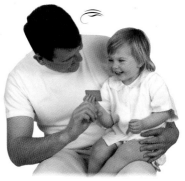

EVE ROGANS

ELEMENT

SHAFTESBURY, DORSET • ROCKPORT, MASSACHUSETTS • MELBOURNE, VICTORIA

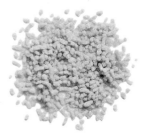

© Element Books Limited 1997

First published
in Great Britain in
1997 by
ELEMENT BOOKS LIMITED
Shaftesbury, Dorset, SP7 9BP

Published in the USA in 1997 by
ELEMENT BOOKS INC
PO Box 830, Rockport, MA 01966

Published in Australia in 1997 by
ELEMENT BOOKS
and distributed by
PENGUIN AUSTRALIA LTD
487 Maroondah Highway, Ringwood,
Victoria 3134

NOTE FROM THE PUBLISHER
Any information given in this book is
not intended to be taken as a replacement
for medical advice. Any person with a
condition requiring medical attention
should consult a qualified practitioner
or therapist.

Designed and created with
The Bridgewater Book Company Ltd

ELEMENT BOOKS LIMITED
Editorial Director Julia McCutchen
Managing Editor Caro Ness
Project Editor Allie West
Production Director Roger Lane
Production Sarah Golden

THE BRIDGEWATER BOOK COMPANY
Art Director Kevin Knight
Designers Andrew Milne, Jane Lanaway
Managing Editor Anne Townley
Project Co-ordinator Fiona Corbridge
Page Layout Chris Lanaway
Picture Research Lynda Marshall
Three-dimensional Models Mark Jamieson
Photography Ian Parsons, Guy Ryecart
Illustrations Andrew Milne, Pip Adams,
Lindsey Tai

Text consultants BOOK CREATION SERVICES LTD
Series Editor Karen Sullivan

Printed and bound by Dai Nippon, Hong Kong

British Library Cataloguing in
Publication data available

Library of Congress Cataloging
in Publication data available

ISBN 1–86204–105–9

The publishers wish to thank the following for the
use of pictures: A–Z Botanical Collection Ltd,
Bridgeman Art Library, e. t. archive, Harry
Smith Collection, Science Photo Library,
Werner Forman Archive, and Zefa.

Special thanks go to:
Stephen Sparshatt and Carys Lecrass
for help with photography

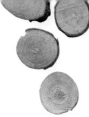

Contents

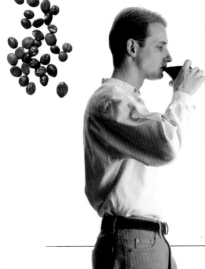

What is Chinese medicine?

CHINESE MEDICINE *is a system of diagnosis and complete healthcare based on a holistic ("whole") understanding of our bodies, minds, and spirits, in conjunction with the universe. It embraces the spiritual insights of "Taoism," which is a Chinese philosophical system that relies on our harmonious interaction with the environment.*

ABOVE *The teachings of the Chinese sage, Confucius, are still studied today.*

Over the last 20 years, Chinese medicine has become increasingly popular in the West.

Acupuncture was the first Chinese therapy to gain widespread acceptance among those seeking treatment, following a marked trend towards alternatives to the orthodox medical systems. People suffering from conditions such as backache and stress wanted something other than pills for chronic problems, and acupuncture offered a safe and effective option.

Over the last decade Chinese herbal medicine has become well known in Britain and the U.S., where it has received particular acclaim for the successful treatment of skin disorders among the Western medical establishments.

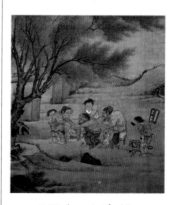

ABOVE *A country physician applying the Chinese cure of moxibustion to a patient's back.*

TRADITIONAL CHINESE MEDICINE (T.C.M.)

Chinese medicine is an ancient system that has evolved over more than two thousand years. It is based on the philosophy of a very different civilization to our own, and it has therefore developed its own way of perceiving the body and the processes of illness.

Chinese medicine uses terminology that Westerners will find strange – such as diseases being caused by Dampness, Wind, or Heat. Illness is not classified in terms of the same body systems that we use in Western medicine, such as the nervous system or the endocrine system. However, Chinese medicine does successfully treat neurological or endocrine disorders, and deals with bacteria it does not recognize.

RIGHT *Meditation is recommended to strengthen the spirit.*

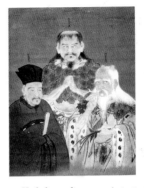

ABOVE *Herbal remedies are an important part of traditional Chinese medicine.*

Traditional Chinese medicine views the body as a whole and sees disease in terms of patterns of disharmony. The treatments try to bring the person back into balance and consequently restore the harmony of health. As well as acupuncture and herbal remedies, treatments include those practices that can easily be incorporated into everyday life, such as diet, meditation, and exercise.

A short history

HERBAL FORMULAE *have been transcribed in China since the 3rd century* B.C.E. *The fundamental book of Chinese medicine, the* Yellow Emperor's Inner Classic, *was compiled in the 1st century* C.E., *but the basis of the system was well in place by then. Early acupuncture was carried out with sharpened fragments of bone.*

ABOVE **The Chinese have recorded herbal formulae for centuries.**

Over the centuries, leading physicians have added many thousands of herbal and acupuncture formulae to the established theories as the practice has developed. The *Imperial Grace Formulary* of the Tai Pang Era, which was compiled around 985C.E, contains 16,834 herbal entries in one volume.

The *Divine Husbandman's Classic of the Materia Medica* is another ancient work with specific emphasis on herbal remedies – and its herbal combinations are still in use today. Indeed, much of today's practice of Chinese medicine reflects traditions that have developed over the course of 3,000 years.

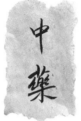

ABOVE **The character for Chinese medicine.**

TWIN PHILOSOPHIES

Chinese medicine is based on the twin philosophies of Yin and Yang (the dual forces in the universe that are forever changing), and the Five Phases or Elements of Water, Fire, Wood, Metal, and Earth. These Elements represent the ancient view of the changing seasons and the way humans fit into them. If we are not in harmony with the movements of nature, we become ill and if Yin and Yang are out of balance, illness is the inevitable result.

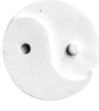

ABOVE **The symbol for Yin and Yang represents them as interdependent.**

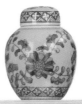
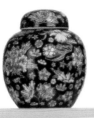

HERBAL FORMULAE

The early herbal formulae were very simple and elegant. The later ones are much more complicated. Both have their strengths and weaknesses.

A Chinese herbal practitioner will diagnose the patient's pattern of disharmony, take the tried and tested prescription which is closest to that patient's pattern, and add or subtract herbs to make it more suitable for that individual. Herbs are seldom used singly: they are usually combined in prescriptions containing between 5 and 15 substances.

DONG GUA PI

BAI ZHI

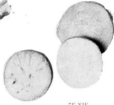

ABOVE **Herb storage jars. Each herb has different qualities and properties.**

ZE XIE

SHU DI HUANG

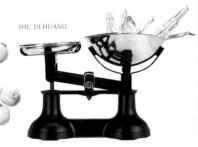

LIAN ZI

ABOVE AND RIGHT
Each prescription is made up of many different ingredients, some of which are shown here.

OU JIE

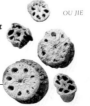

9

Setting the scene

CHINESE MEDICINE *is holistic – meaning that no single part of an individual or a condition can be understood except in its relation to the whole. Western medicine focuses on a specific cause for each disease, and when it isolates that cause or agent, it tries to control or destroy it. Chinese medicine is also concerned with the cause, but more so with the patient's physiological and psychological response to disease as a whole.*

ABOVE **The dragon is believed to affect energy flow.**

YIN AND YANG TREATMENTS

In the Chinese philosophy of the complementary opposites Yin and Yang, acupuncture is considered Yang, because it moves from the outside in, while herbalism is Yin because it works from the inside out. Herbalism can support acupuncture treatment, or it may be used on its own. Conditions such as viral infections and blood disorders (anemia or menstrual problems), may be better suited to herbal treatment than to acupuncture. Herbs are also used to strengthen those people who are too weak to have acupuncture.

YIN YANG SYMBOL

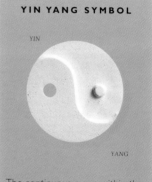

YIN

YANG

The continuous curve within the Yin Yang symbol indicates that Yin and Yang are continuously changing from one to the other. The dot from the opposite half shows that there is always a seed of one side in the other.

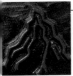

YIN

YANG

THE THEORY OF YIN AND YANG

Yin and Yang are labels used to explain the ongoing process of natural change; for example, Yin inhalation is followed by Yang exhalation. All things have a Yin viewpoint and a Yang viewpoint.

• Everything is relative – a Cold Yin illness may have some of the aspects of Yang such as sharp, forceful contractions.

• Yin and Yang depend on each other – Yang activity is nourished by Yin physical form.

• Yin and Yang control each other – if Yin is in excess, Yang will be weak. A Cold-Damp illness (*see page 30–31*) will make a patient still and inactive.

• Good health means the proportions of Yin and Yang are relatively balanced. Illness means that these proportions are unequal. Changes in the proportions can also be too dramatic – fever and sweat may transform into sudden shock and cold.

BELOW *Complementary aspects of Yin and Yang.*

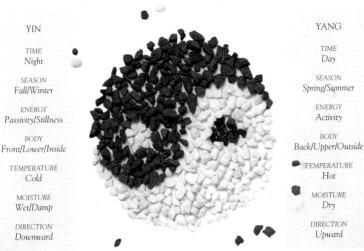

YIN	YANG
TIME *Night*	TIME *Day*
SEASON *Fall/Winter*	SEASON *Spring/Summer*
ENERGY *Passivity/Stillness*	ENERGY *Activity*
BODY *Front/Lower/Inside*	BODY *Back/Upper/Outside*
TEMPERATURE *Cold*	TEMPERATURE *Hot*
MOISTURE *Wet/Damp*	MOISTURE *Dry*
DIRECTION *Downward*	DIRECTION *Upward*

The human body

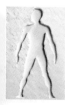

ABOVE **Chi**
inhabits the
whole body.

THE CHINESE *view the human body as an energy system,*
made up of different, interacting substances. These are
Chi, Jing, Body Fluids, and Shen. Chi is the life force that
permeates the whole body. Jing is the essence of life. Blood
(as well as its usual meaning) is a substance that nourishes
the body and the Shen. Body Fluids moisten and lubricate
the body. Shen is the mental or spiritual side of a person.

Chi is also important to
health because it is the
energy that binds Yin and Yang.
Together with Blood and
moisture, it flows around the
body in channels called

meridians keeping us alive and
healthy. When Chi flows freely,
Yin, Yang, and the whole person
are in balance. But when Chi is
unbalanced, stagnant, or blocked,
it can lead to illness.

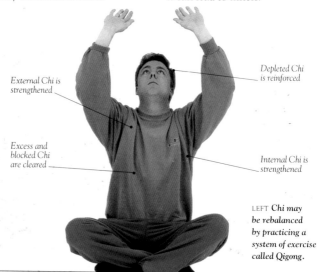

External Chi is
strengthened

Excess and
blocked Chi
are cleared

Depleted Chi
is reinforced

Internal Chi is
strengthened

LEFT **Chi may**
be rebalanced
by practicing a
system of exercise
called Qigong.

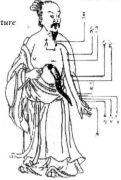

RIGHT *Acupuncture points along the Lung meridian.*

MERIDIANS

• Meridians are the channels or pathways along which Chi flows through the organs and body parts, adjusting and harmonizing their activity.

• Most acupuncture points are sited along these channels, and most herbs prescribed by a Chinese physician will enter one or more of the meridian pathways.

• There are 12 main meridians, each of which corresponds to the 12 main organs in the body. Each is bilateral – with an identical partner on the other side of the body.

• There are six extra meridians and other minor meridians called *Luo* meridians.

FUNCTIONS OF CHI

• Chi directs the systems in the body (blood, nervous, and lymphatic).

• It is the source of movement and growth.

• It protects the body from Outside Pernicious Influences (OPI) such as viruses and bacteria, and combats them if they do penetrate.

• It transforms food into the bodily substances of blood, tears, sweat, and urine.

• It keeps everything in: organs in their proper place, blood in vessels. It also prevents excessive loss of sweat.

• Chi warms the body.

• It is used to describe the functions of any organ. In disease, Lung Chi may be weak, or Liver Chi may be blocked.

ORIGINS OF CHI

• According to T.C.M., prenatal Chi or "genetic energy" (Yuan Chi) from our parents is stored in the kidneys, and makes up part of our energy levels.

• Grain Chi (Gu Chi) is energy released from the breakdown and digestion of food.

• Natural Air Chi (Kong Chi) enters our bodies through our lungs, in the air we breathe.

13

THE MERIDIAN THEORY OF ILLNESS

Meridian theory assumes that any disorder that occurs within a meridian, or within that meridian's connecting organ, will cause disharmony along the whole course of that meridian channel.

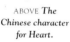

ABOVE *The Chinese character for Heart.*

The Stomach meridian, for example, runs from the second toe, up the outside of the legs, through the abdomen, the teeth and jaw, right up to the eye. This means that toothache

TYPES OF MERIDIAN

- **YIN MERIDIANS**
Kidney, Liver, Spleen, Heart, Lungs, and Pericardium (an "organ" for these purposes).
- **YANG MERIDIANS**
Bladder, Gall Bladder, Stomach, Small Intestine, Large Intestine, and the Triple Burner (a mechanism which regulates the overall body temperature, and the Upper, Middle, and Lower parts (Jiaos) of the body).

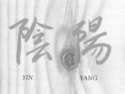

YIN   YANG

ABOVE *The Chinese characters for Yin and Yang*

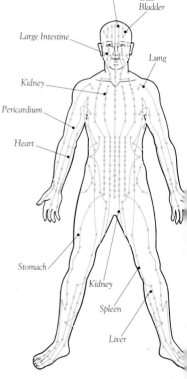

Bladder

Gall Bladder

Large Intestine

Lung

Kidney

Pericardium

Heart

Stomach

Kidney

Spleen

Liver

may be caused by a disorder along any part of the Stomach meridian and will be treated via that channel. For example, Stomach Fire is a disharmony that may include toothache as one of its symptoms.

BELOW *Meridians are invisible channels along which Chi flows around the body. There are 12 main meridians.*

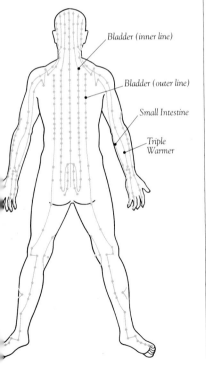

Bladder (inner line)

Bladder (outer line)

Small Intestine

Triple Warmer

DISHARMONY CAUSES ILLNESS

In illness, different meridians exhibit different tendencies to disharmony. For example, the Spleen has a tendency to deficiency causing Damp. This creates symptoms such as diarrhea or lassitude (tiredness). The Liver, on the other hand, has a tendency towards Rising Yang, creating sore, red eyes, migraines, and high blood-pressure. It is disharmonies such as these that Chinese herbal medicine addresses.

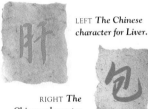

LEFT *The Chinese character for Liver.*

RIGHT *The Chinese character for Pericardium.*

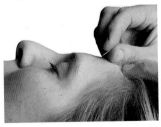

ABOVE *Acupunture removes obstructions along the invisible channels of the body.*

Consulting a Chinese herbalist

When you consult a Chinese herbalist, he or she will ask you in detail about your presenting condition – when it first appeared, the symptoms, and what makes it worse or better. The herbalist will then ask about your past medical history, your lifestyle, and your general health.

LEFT **A prescription may contain a complex assortment of herbs.**

THE CONSULTATION

Be prepared to answer questions on the following subjects.
- Your appetite, diet, digestion, stools, and urination.
- Your sleep patterns.
- Whether you suffer from any pain, such as headaches or backache.
- Whether you have problems with your ears, nose, or throat.
- Your intake of drugs, alcohol, and nicotine.
- Your body temperature (whether you are more of a "cold" or "hot" person).
- Your circulation.
- Your levels of perspiration.
- Your energy levels, mental and emotional states.

- Gynecology – menstruation, pregnancies, menopause.

Finally, your practitioner will take both radial (wrist) pulses and look at your tongue in detail.

BELOW **Each wrist is thought to contain six pulses.**

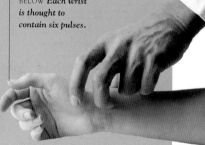

DIAGNOSIS

The herbalist will make a diagnosis according to Chinese principles and will probably search through reference books to find the herbal prescription most suited to your condition. Your practitioner will write a prescription that is individual to you, and which will include anything from 4 to 20 herbs with their dosages in ounces, grams, or in qian (a Chinese measurement).

The names of the herbs will be in English, Latin, Pin-Yin (anglicized Chinese), or in Chinese characters. Your practitioner will then make up the prescription for you or refer you to a herbal supplier to have it made up.

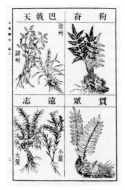

ABOVE *An early book listing plants and their applications.*

FINDING A HERBALIST

You can get in touch with a registered Chinese herbalist by consulting the relevant professional body in your area. For suggestions see page 59.

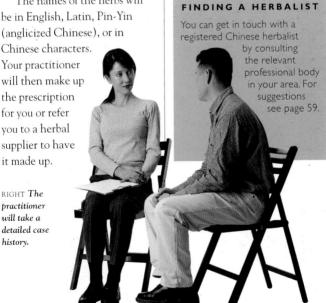

RIGHT *The practitioner will take a detailed case history.*

TREATMENT

Treatment generally means taking herbs two or three times a day until the problem has been rectified. Remedies can take the form of a decoction (made by boiling a package of dried herbs in water), powders (also boiled in water and drunk), tinctures (drink only in a prescribed dose), or pills.

Following the initial consultation, which can take anything up to an hour and a half, you will need to see your practitioner once a week or every two weeks. This is so that the prescription can be adjusted as your symptoms change and you begin to get well.

You may experience slight nausea, diarrhea, or digestive upset as your system becomes used to the herbs, but this is normal and usually a good sign. If your symptoms become too uncomfortable, you can halve the dosage, building it up to the correct dosage over time. Your practitioner may add more digestive herbs to make the remedy more tolerable.

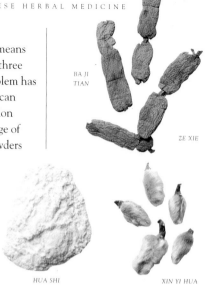

BA JI TIAN

ZE XIE

HUA SHI

XIN YI HUA

When treatment is well under way, you may see or even telephone your practitioner once a month in order to report on progress. Herbal medicines should not be taken for more than 30 days without review.

CAUTION

Do not prepare your own remedies except under the instructions of a qualified herbalist.

ABOVE AND RIGHT
Chinese medicine uses a wide variety of animal, plant and mineral sources. These are a few of the thousands of remedies available.

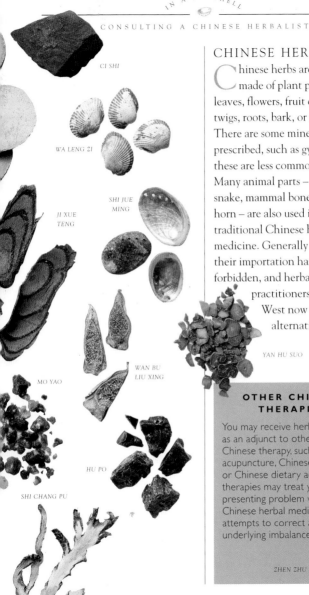

CI SHI

WA LENG ZI

SHI JUE MING

JI XUE TENG

WAN BU LIU XING

MO YAO

HU PO

SHI CHANG PU

YAN HU SUO

CHINESE HERBS

Chinese herbs are mostly made of plant parts – leaves, flowers, fruit or fruit peel, twigs, roots, bark, or fungus. There are some minerals that are prescribed, such as gypsum, but these are less commonly used. Many animal parts – such as snake, mammal bones, or deer horn – are also used in traditional Chinese herbal medicine. Generally however, their importation has been forbidden, and herbal practitioners in the West now use alternatives.

OTHER CHINESE THERAPIES

You may receive herbal medicine as an adjunct to other forms of Chinese therapy, such as acupuncture, Chinese massage, or Chinese dietary advice. These therapies may treat your presenting problem while Chinese herbal medicine attempts to correct a long-term underlying imbalance.

ZHEN ZHU MU

Herbal theory

Herbs are categorized according to taste and temperature. Tastes are acrid, sweet, bitter, sour, salty, and bland. Temperatures are Hot, Cold, Warm, Cool, Neutral, and varying degrees between.

Hot diseases must be treated with cooling herbs, though it is important not to cool too much, or the body may try to compensate by warming up again. Cold diseases must be treated with heating herbs, and the same warning applies.

Prescriptions include herbs that will prevent the balance from swinging too far in the other direction, and herbs that will strengthen the digestion in order that the herbs are absorbed more effectively.

Chen Pi regulates Chi

Fu Ling drains Damp

Sheng Di Huang nourishes the Blood

Gui Zhi expels Cold

SHENG DI HUANG
Sweet, bitter, cold

RIGHT **The actions of some Chinese herbs.**

HERBS AND
THEIR PROPERTIES

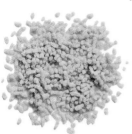

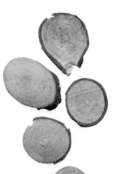

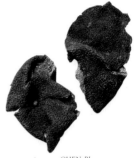

CHEN PI
*Acrid, bitter, warm,
fragrant*

REN SHEN
*Sweet, slightly bitter,
slightly warm*

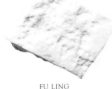

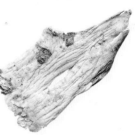

GUI ZHI
Acrid, sweet, warm

FU LING
Sweet, bland, neutral

JIE GENG
Bitter, acrid, neutral

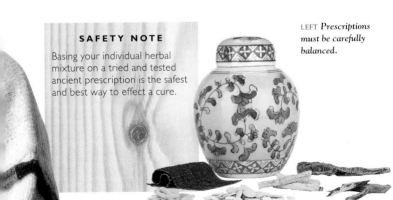

SAFETY NOTE

Basing your individual herbal
mixture on a tried and tested
ancient prescription is the safest
and best way to effect a cure.

LEFT *Prescriptions
must be carefully
balanced.*

Preparations

THERE ARE *many different ways of taking herbs. Individual herbs can be added to foods or taken as a tea, but Chinese herbs are rarely taken singly — they correct imbalance much more effectively in a composite prescription formulated to individual needs.*

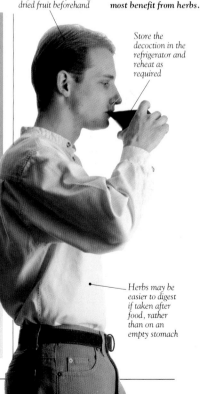

ABOVE **Herbs are boiled in water and strained to make a decoction.**

If you find the taste unpleasant, try eating dried fruit beforehand

BELOW **A decoction allows you to derive the most benefit from herbs.**

Store the decoction in the refrigerator and reheat as required

SYRUPS

• Patent remedies, mainly for coughs, or children's tonics.

TINCTURES

• Herbs suspended in a solution of alcohol.
• One teaspoon (5ml) of liquid taken two to three times a day.
• Tinctures are easier on the palate, but are not as powerful as decoctions or powders.

HERBS

The taste of herbs may seem strange at first but you will soon become accustomed to the unique flavors. Many people grow to enjoy them.

Keep cooked herbs in the refrigerator.

Herbs may be easier to digest if taken after food, rather than on an empty stomach

POWDERS

• Powders are not considered to be as potent as decoctions.
• One teaspoonful (5ml) of cooked, freeze-dried, powdered herbs is taken two to three times a day. It is mixed with a little cold water to a paste, and a little boiling water is then added.
• Powders are somewhat unpalatable but easy and effective.
• Powders are easier to prepare for consumption than decoctions.

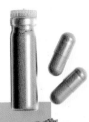

RIGHT *Herbs may be dried and ground into powders.*

PLASTERS

• Used for rheumatic ailments (Wind-Damp – see page 30–31); very effective for relieving local pain and stiffness.

ABOVE *Tinctures are stored in glass bottles.*

BELOW *Yunnan Pai Yao capsules, used to treat insect bites.*

DECOCTIONS

• Packets of dried herbs are boiled in a large pot of boiling water for around thirty minutes, until they are reduced to about two cups.
• Decoctions are often strained and boiled again to last a day or two.
• They smell worse than they taste!

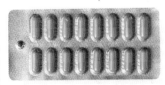

PILLS

• Sold as patent remedies – prescriptions made to a set formula.
• Easy to swallow, but you have to take a lot more than is usual with Western drugs (sometimes eight tablets at a time).

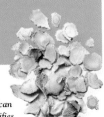

RIGHT *American Ren Shen tonifies Yin Chi.*

23

Patent herbal preparations

PATENT FORMULA
IN PILL FORM

LOQUAT COUGH
POWDER

PATENT HERBAL *preparations are sold as over-the-counter remedies for conditions as wide ranging as colds and influenza, coughs and phlegm, strept (streptococcal) throat infections, rheumatic ailments, and pain and bruising from trauma.*

Patent remedies used for anything other than the above must be diagnosed by a herbal practitioner. In particular, Chinese herbal tonics must be individually prescribed. They will be made up to tonify either Chi, Blood, Yin, or Yang.

Patent remedies used over a long period of time must be prescribed by qualified herbal practitioners. Tonics may be given to help with underlying problems, for instance in the elderly, while more immediate complaints are being dealt with.

ABOVE AND LEFT **Classic formulae, which have proved successful over centuries, are manufactured as patent remedies.**

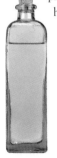

HERBAL TONIC

SAFETY NOTE

If herbs are prescribed over a long period of time, it is important that the practitioner pays particular attention to any liver or kidney symptoms which arise during the course of treatment. Toxic herbs have been banned in most Western countries. However, a few individuals may experience idiosyncratic reactions to certain herbs. Regular liver function tests are sometimes advised by practitioners, but their value is still a matter of debate.

CHILDREN AND BABIES

Chinese herbal medicine can be very effective for children and babies. Children's dosages are usually half or a quarter of those for adults. There are ways of encouraging children to take the herbs, either by involving them in the preparation of the prescription, or by sweetening it with honey, or by offering a cookie afterwards! There are certain herbal powders especially formulated for babies.

BELOW LEFT *The prospect of a sweet reward may make the medicine more appealing.*

Try to make medicine-taking fun!

Offer a cookie afterwards

PREGNANCY

Many herbs are expressly forbidden in pregnancy; others are especially good for pregnant women. There are several which may help to prevent miscarriage. If you are pregnant, tell your practitioner, and only take herbs he or she has prescribed. Do not attempt to treat yourself with patent remedies.

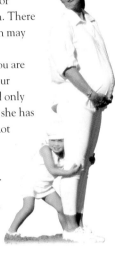

RIGHT *As with all medical treatments, great care should be exercised during pregnancy.*

CAUTION

Some patent remedies may still contain animal products. Make sure the remedy you are purchasing does not, as they are now illegal in most Western countries. Always go to a reputable practitioner or pharmacy for your herbs.

Some patent remedies for insomnia and mental disturbance contain mineral substances such as oyster shell or magnetite. In excess, these can cause indigestion. Use these for a limited period of time only.

Tonics must not be taken during an episode of colds or influenza, as they tend to drive Wind deeper into the body. Chi tonics slightly stagnate energy and may therefore cause abdominal bloating if not properly prescribed.

Chinese medical terminology

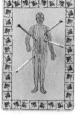

ABOVE *Acupuncture points are sited along meridian paths.*

THIS SECTION *is a glossary, which will provide you with a general understanding of the herbs' functions in terms of Chinese medical philosophy. It clarifies the meaning of the organs in T.C.M., gives details about the basic terms used, explains what the taste of a herb involves, and gives the causes of various diseases.*

ORGANS (AND THEIR CORRESPONDING CHANNELS)

The concept of the organs (Tsang Fu) in Traditional Chinese Medicine is radically different from that in the West. When Chinese physicians talk about a particular organ, they are not usually talking about the physical structure of that organ, but a complex series of functions that it is seen to perform in the body. When the names of organs, body parts, or actions begin with a capital letter, it implies the Chinese concepts and functions of those organs or body parts, rather than merely the physical organ itself. For example, the

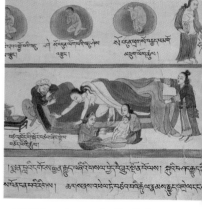

ABOVE *An ancient text detailing birth and the reproductive system.*

Kidney meridian would govern the function of everything along that meridian, including the kidneys themselves.

Kidneys

The Kidneys store Jing (genetic energy), which rules birth, growth, development, and reproduction. The Kidney rules the bones, opens into the ears, and manifests itself in the hair. It rules the Water (all the fluids in the body) and receives and holds Chi from the Lungs.

Spleen

The Spleen rules the absorption of food and drink, helping to transport the products to different parts of the body. The Spleen is the main digestive organ in T.C.M. It rules the muscles, limbs, and the Blood. It holds up the organs, opens into the mouth, and shows in the lips. When the spleen is in disharmony it may cause an accumulation of fluids, creating Damp and edema in the body.

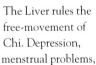

ABOVE *The Chinese character for Spleen.*

Liver

The Liver rules the free-movement of Chi. Depression, menstrual problems, and cramp are caused by Liver malfunctions. The Liver stores the Blood, opens into the eyes, and manifests in the nails. When the Liver clogs up with Damp-Heat, hepatitis results.

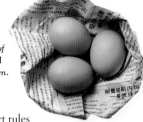

RIGHT *The absorption of food is ruled by the Spleen.*

Heart

The Heart rules the Blood and blood vessels, and stores the Shen (spirit). If the Shen is harmonious, the mind is peaceful; if it is disturbed, the mind is restless, causing insomnia and poor memory. The Heart shows in the complexion and opens into the tongue – stuttering or poor speech is often a Heart problem.

ABOVE *The Chinese character for Liver.*

Lungs

The Lungs rule Chi and the exterior of the body, and govern respiration. The Lungs open into the nose and manifest in the body hair. Respiratory problems, colds, and dry skin are treated via the Lungs.

Pericardium

The Pericardium is traditionally considered to protect the Heart from attack by infectious diseases. Its functions are similar to those of the Heart, but it has a distinct meridian.

ABOVE *The Chinese character for Heart.*

Bladder

The Bladder receives, stores, and transforms fluids before they are excreted as urine. Deficiency of Kidney Yang may cause bed-wetting, incontinence, and other problems. Stagnation of the free-flow of water may result in Damp accumulating in the Bladder, leading to a build-up of Damp-Heat (cystitis).

Stomach

Known as "the Sea of Food and Water," the Stomach separates food and drink into "pure" and "impure." The pure part goes to the Spleen for further distribution, the impure goes down to the Small Intestines, then to the Large Intestines or Bladder. If the descending power of the Stomach is disturbed, belching, epigastric (upper abdominal) pain, and hiccups will result.

Gall Bladder

The Gall Bladder stores bile and is very closely related to the Liver. Both the Gall Bladder and the Liver are often involved in hepatitis, cholecystitis (inflammation of the gall bladder) and gallstones. Emotionally, both are characterized by anger and irritability.

BASIC TERMS

Chi

Life force or vital energy. When Chi comes together, it forms the physical body; when it disperses, it becomes the driving force behind all the processes in the

LEFT *External heat is drying and causes inflamed skin.*

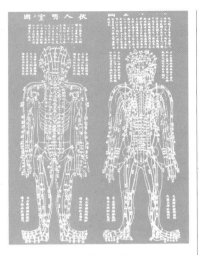

ABOVE *The meridian system consists of 12 main channels.*

body. It shows itself in the different functions it performs. Chi deficiency symptoms include lethargy and lack of desire to move. "Chi deficiency" may also be used to describe a particular organ unable to perform its functions.

Blood
A more Yin, dense form of Chi, which nourishes and moistens the body.

Blood deficiency
When the body is insufficiently nourished by the Blood, it is characterized by a pale face, dizziness, and dry skin. Blood deficiency can also affect particular organs – deficient Heart Blood causes palpitations.

Yang deficiency
A further progression of Chi deficiency, which nearly always includes Cold symptoms.

Yin deficiency
Means the Yang will not be controlled and will rise up and outward, causing fluids to leak out at night, manifesting as night sweats and dry skin.

Tonify
To increase the power or the amount of something (for example Chi, Yang, or Yin) in a particular meridian, when it is deficient or lacking.

Disperse/Sedate
To help break up Stagnant Chi or Blood, or to decrease the power of something that is in excess in a particular meridian – for example Yin or Chi.

ABOVE *The Chinese character for Pericardium.*

Harmonize

Mainly refers to herbs that affect the Liver when it loses its function of harmonizing the Chi and Blood in the body.

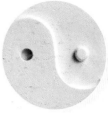

RIGHT *Yin and Yang are central to Chinese medicine.*

TASTES

In T.C.M., the taste of a herb partly determines its therapeutic function.

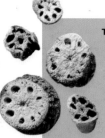

OU JIE

- **Acrid**
Disperses and moves Chi. Mainly affects the Lungs.

- **Sweet**
Tonifies, harmonizes, and sometimes moistens. Mainly affects the Spleen.

- **Bitter**
Drains and dries. Mainly affects the Heart.

- **Sour**
Prevents or reverses the abnormal leakage of fluids and energy. Mainly affects the Liver.

- **Salty**
Purges the bowels and softens. Mainly affects the Kidneys.

- **Bland**
Leeches out Dampness and promotes urination. This helps both the Spleen and the Kidneys.

SOME CAUSES OF DISEASE

Wind

External Wind refers to a disease caused by a viral or bacterial infection. It is usually accompanied by Cold (feeling cold), Heat (fever) or Damp (nausea and vomiting). Internal Wind is associated with spasms, tremors, itching, stroke, and numbness. Deficiency of the Liver is often a cause of Internal Wind.

CHEN PI

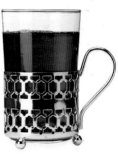

ABOVE *A decoction is a beneficial way of taking herbs.*

Cold

Any disease where the person feels cold, or is made worse by cold, is a Yin disease. Cold slows the circulation in the meridians, so that the Chi is unable to penetrate, resulting in pain.

Heat/Fire

Characterized by signs such as high fever, red face, thirst, scanty, dark urine, rapid pulse, hemorrhaging, and red skin eruptions. This is a Yang-type disease.

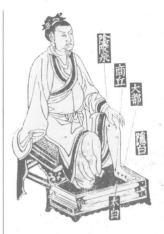

ABOVE *The Spleen and Liver meridians are located on the leg.*

Damp

Characterized by symptoms that are wet, heavy, and slow. This is a Yin-type disease. It can be caused by living in damp surroundings or eating Damp-producing foods in excess (dairy products, for instance). Distinguished by heavy diarrhea, vaginal discharge, cloudy urine, soreness in the joints, dull pain, coated tongue. The Spleen is the organ most affected by Dampness.

Phlegm

Phlegm is a progression of Damp, and is usually a more chronic deficiency of the Spleen, Lungs,

and Kidney Yang. If it combines with Wind, it may result in facial paralysis, stroke, or epilepsy.

Dryness

Associated with dry nostrils, lips, dry skin, and constipation. External Dryness often interferes with the functions of the Lungs. Smoking cigarettes puts Dry Heat into the Lungs, an organ that needs moisture to function properly.

LICORICE LEAVES

Chinese herbs

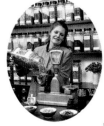

CHINESE HERBS *are hardly ever used singly – they are mainly used in combination with other herbs to make a balanced prescription. The herbs on the following pages are some of the most commonly prescribed. Each herb has a particular range of dosages assigned to it. Do not try to treat yourself without the advice of a qualified herbalist, who will advise you of the correct proportions.*

ABOVE *Weighing out supplies at a herbal pharmacy.*

RIGHT *Chinese herbs are used to treat all areas of the body by rebalancing Chi, Yin, and Yang along the meridian pathways.*

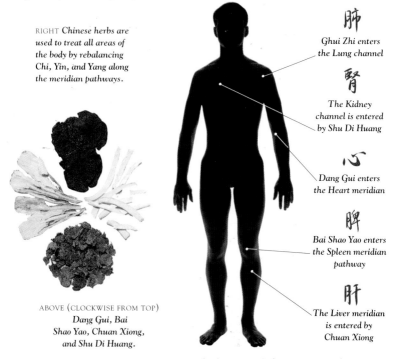

肺

Ghui Zhi enters the Lung channel

腎

The Kidney channel is entered by Shu Di Huang

心

Dang Gui enters the Heart meridian

脾

Bai Shao Yao enters the Spleen meridian pathway

肝

The Liver meridian is entered by Chuan Xiong

ABOVE (CLOCKWISE FROM TOP) *Dang Gui, Bai Shao Yao, Chuan Xiong, and Shu Di Huang.*

Sheng Di Huang

RADIX REHMANNIA GLUTINOSA
Chinese Foxglove Root

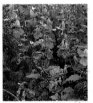

RIGHT *A field of Chinese foxgloves, source of Sheng Di Huang.*

PROPERTIES
Sweet, Bitter, and Cold

CHANNELS ENTERED
Heart, Liver, and Kidney

Sheng Di Huang is a very moistening, as well as cooling, herb. Therefore it is used in illnesses where there is fever or where reduced fluids in the body have caused thirst, irritability, and a scarlet tongue. It is also used, often with Bai Shao, when Heat in the Blood level causes hemorrhage, such as bloody urine, nosebleeds, or vomiting of blood. Sheng Di Huang may be used to treat diabetes and also helps the body to replace fluids. Because it is moist, it needs digestive herbs with it to avoid causing Dampness in the digestive system. It must not be used if there is Phlegm.

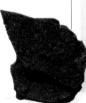

FUNCTIONS AND USES

Clears Heat and cools the Blood – used in all conditions where there is a very high fever, thirst, and a scarlet tongue. Also in hemorrhage when Heat enters the Blood level (according to T.C.M.).

◆

Nourishes the Yin and generates fluids – useful for low-grade long-term fever with dry mouth, constipation, and night sweats.

◆

Cools Heart Fire blazing – mouth and tongue ulcers, irritability, and insomnia.

◆

Treats Wasting-Thirsting syndrome, for example, diabetes.

SHENG DI HUANG

CHINESE HERBAL MEDICINE

Gan Jiang

ZINGIBER OFFICINALE
Dried Ginger Root

PROPERTIES
Acrid, Hot

CHANNELS ENTERED
Spleen, Stomach, Lung, and Kidney

The most important action of Gan Jiang is its ability to treat Cold-deficient conditions – this includes a thin pulse, white tongue, and other Cold symptoms. It is a valuable herb as it not only warms the Middle area (Spleen and Stomach) but also treats Lung and Kidney symptoms. It is contraindicated in Deficient Yin patterns with Heat signs or in Hot bleeding, and must be used with caution during pregnancy.

RIGHT **Fresh ginger root has many culinary uses, as well as medical applications.**

FUNCTIONS AND USES

Warms the Middle and expels Cold – warms the Spleen and Stomach. For lack of appetite, cold limbs, diarrhea, vomiting, and abdominal pain.

◆

Rescues devastated Yang and expels Interior Cold (person in shock, very cold, weak pulse).

◆

Warms the Lungs and transforms Phlegm – for Cold Lung patterns with thin, watery sputum.

◆

Warms the channels and stops hemorrhage of the Cold-deficient type; for example, chronic, fairly pale bleeding with other Cold and Deficient symptoms.

Huo Ma Ren

CANNABIS SATIVA
Marijuana Seeds

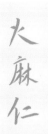

PROPERTIES
Sweet,
Neutral

CHANNELS ENTERED
Spleen,
Stomach,
and Large
Intestine

Huo Ma Ren are ungerminated cannabis seeds and, as such, do not have the effects that smoking cannabis leaves or resin has! They must be ground up in a pestle and mortar before boiling. Huo Ma Ren is widely used as a gentle moistening herb to treat constipation, for which it is combined with Dang Gui and Sheng Di Huang in the herbal pill Run Chang Wan. Overdosage can be the cause of nausea and vomiting, so it is advisable to avoid large doses.

FUNCTIONS AND USES

Moistens and nourishes the Intestines – used for constipation, particularly in the elderly, after childbirth, or in Deficient Blood cases.

◆

Nourishes the Yin – mildly tonifies the Yin, but mainly used for Yin-deficient (fluid-deficient) constipation.

◆

Clears Heat and promotes healing of sores – used externally for sores and ulcers.

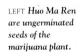

LEFT *Huo Ma Ren are ungerminated seeds of the marijuana plant.*

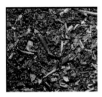

HUO XIANG

Huo Xiang

HERBA AGASTACHES SEU POGOSTEMI
Wrinkled Giant Hyssop/Patchouli

PROPERTIES
Acrid, Slightly
Warm

**CHANNELS
ENTERED**
Lung, Spleen,
and Stomach

Huo Xiang is used when Dampness has created internal obstruction, to help the Spleen recover its function of transporting and transforming food around the body. It is the Emperor herb (main herb) in the patent formula Huo Xiang Zheng Chi Wan, which is used for gastric influenza.

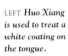

LEFT *Huo Xiang is used to treat a white coating on the tongue.*

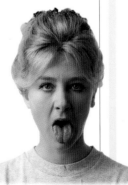

FUNCTIONS AND USES

Transforms Dampness – abdominal or epigastric (below the ribs) bloating, nausea, fatigue, lack of appetite, and moist white coating on the tongue.

◆

Harmonizes the Middle area and stops vomiting. May also be used for morning sickness.

◆

Releases the exterior and expels Dampness – as in gastric influenza.

CAUTION

No herbs used for getting rid of Damp (shown by a thick tongue coating or by the presence of phlegm) may be used in Deficient Yin with Heat signs conditions, which are shown by a peeled tongue.

Fu Ling

PORIA COCOS

Tuckahoe/Hoelen or Bread Root

FU LING

PROPERTIES
Sweet, Bland,
Neutral

**CHANNELS
ENTERED**
Heart, Spleen,
and Lung

Fu Ling is a widely used fungus as it strengthens the Spleen and gets rid of Dampness (a common condition in a cold, damp climate such as that in the U.K.) and it therefore helps the digestion. It is a main ingredient in the Chi-strengthening prescription Liu Jun Zi Wan (the Four Gentlemen decoction). It is also essential in the Yin-tonifying prescription Liu Wei di Huang Wan, to help balance the main Yin-tonifying herbs which might make the patient too moist, causing digestive problems as a result. The herb has few contraindications and is safe for most people to use.

FUNCTIONS AND USES

Promotes urination and leeches out Dampness. For difficult urination, diarrhea, or edema (water retention).

Strengthens the Spleen and harmonizes the Middle area. For loss of appetite, diarrhea, or bloating.

Strengthens the Spleen and transforms Phlegm. Phlegm in T.C.M. can also be a cause of heart palpitations, headaches, and dizziness. It always shows a thick greasy coating on the tongue.

Quietens the Heart and calms the spirit. For palpitations, insomnia, or forgetfulness.

LEFT *Fu Ling helps strengthen the Spleen.*

37

Wu Jia Pi

ACANTHOPANAX GRACILISTYLUS
Acanthopanax

Wu Jia Pi is especially good for arthritis, when the Liver and Kidneys are weak. Kidney energy declines as we get older, causing weakness in the tendons and bones, particularly in the legs. As Wu Jia Pi is warming, it treats Cold-Damp conditions where the circulation is obstructed, as in swelling of the legs or stiff knee joints. It can be taken on its own with wine – add either the dried herb or a decoction to the wine. As Wu Jia Pi is drying, use cautiously for Deficient Yin (deficient fluids) with Heat signs.

五加皮

PROPERTIES
Acrid, Warm

CHANNELS ENTERED
Liver and Kidney

FUNCTIONS AND USES

Expels Wind-Dampness and strengthens the sinews and bones. Used for Wind-Cold-Damp arthritis, especially in the elderly.

♦

Transforms Dampness and reduces swelling. Good for difficulty in urinating and edema.

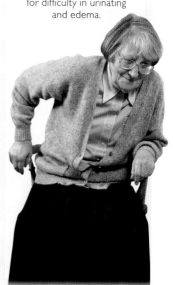

RIGHT **Wu Jia Pi is especially useful for treating arthritis.**

Ban Xia

PINELLIA TERNATA
Pinellia

PROPERTIES
Acrid, Warm,
Poisonous

**CHANNELS
ENTERED**
Spleen and
Stomach

Ban Xia is used for abdominal bloating and nausea caused by Dampness or Phlegm in the Spleen and Stomach. It is often used with Chen Pi, and can be added to prescriptions to avoid nausea. Because it is warming and drying, Ban Xia must be used cautiously in all Heat conditions, where there is Deficient Yin or depleted fluids. In very large amounts, it is somewhat toxic, but can be antidoted by Gian Jiang (a digestive herb).

RIGHT *Ban Xia calms stomach problems. It is useful for morning sickness.*

FUNCTIONS AND USES

Dries Dampness and expels mucus. For coughs with copious amounts of sputum (a Cold condition).

♦

It helps the Spleen to dry out and thereby produce less mucus.

♦

Harmonizes the Stomach and stops vomiting – an important anti-emetic, especially useful during pregnancy.

♦

Reduces lumps and scatters nodules or pain resulting from Phlegm in the chest and goiter.

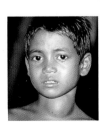

LEFT *Goiter is an enlargement of the thyroid gland, often appearing as a swelling in the neck. Ban Xia can be used in its treatment.*

Jie Geng

RADIX PLATYCODI GRANDIFLORI
Balloon Flower Root/Platycodon

PROPERTIES
Bitter, Acrid, Neutral

CHANNELS ENTERED
Lung

A herb widely used for any Lung problems. As its temperature is average, it can deal with both Hot and Cold, Chi-deficient or Yin-deficient (lack of fluids) nose or throat problems. It is added to many prescriptions to direct other herbs to the upper body. Only contraindicated if the patient is coughing blood (it helps mucus come out, so might make bleeding worse).

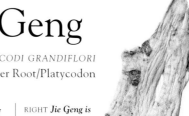

RIGHT *Jie Geng is an ascending herb, influencing the top of the body.*

FUNCTIONS AND USES

Circulates Lung Chi and expels phlegm. Used for a wide variety of coughs, depending on the herbs with which it is combined. Useful for chronic or acute Wind-Heat coughs.

◆

Benefits the throat. For sore throat or loss of voice resulting from a virus or a Yin deficiency with rising Heat symptoms.

◆

Encourages the discharge of pus – especially pus associated with Lung or throat abscesses.

◆

Directs the effects of other herbs to the upper part of the body.

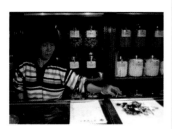

ABOVE *Purchasing Chinese herbs from a specialist supplier.*

Ren Shen

RADIX GINSENG
Panax Ginseng

PROPERTIES
Sweet, Slightly
Bitter, Slightly
Warm

**CHANNELS
ENTERED**
Lung and
Spleen

Ginseng root is a valuable herb (both in financial and functional terms), not only because it takes six to seven years to cultivate, but also because it tonifies both the Chi (effectively combating fatigue) and the Yin (by generating fluid). It is very calming and has a proven effect on stress. As Ginseng is slightly warming, it is contraindicated for Yin deficiency with rising Heat, or for high blood-pressure. As it is so expensive, it is often substituted by Dang Shen in prescriptions.

RIGHT **Ginseng should
not be taken over a
long period, or it can
cause health problems.**

FUNCTIONS AND USES

Strong tonifier of root/ancestral/genetic Chi. Used when a person goes into shock, with shallow respiration, shortness of breath, cold limbs, profuse sweating, and a weak pulse. It can be used by itself.

◆

Tonifies the Lungs and benefits the Chi. For labored breathing, wheezing, and when the Kidneys fail to grasp the Chi from the Lungs; for instance, in asthma when the patient cannot breathe in deeply.

◆

Strengthens the Spleen and tonifies the Stomach. Used for lethargy, lack of appetite, bloating, and diarrhea.

◆

Generates fluid and stops thirst. Useful for diabetes and the aftermath of a fever.

◆

Benefits the Heart Chi and calms the spirit. For palpitations with anxiety, insomnia, forgetfulness, and restlessness.

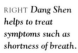

Dang Shen

RADIX CODONOPSIS PILOSULAE
Pilose Asiabell Root

DANG SHEN

Dang Shen does the same work as Ren Shen, but it is weaker and less expensive. The dosage for Dang Shen is therefore higher than for Ren Shen. Dang Shen is used in all Deficient Chi patterns and raises the Yang Chi to lift up any prolapse. It is mainly used for digestive problems and is the Monarch herb (main herb) in the Chi tonic prescription Liu Jun Zi Wan (Four Gentlemen).

PROPERTIES
Raw: Sweet, Neutral;
Fried: Sweet, Warm

CHANNELS ENTERED
All 12 channels – especially Heart, Lung, Spleen, and Stomach

FUNCTIONS AND USES

Tonifies the Middle area, benefits the Chi and strengthens the Stomach and Spleen. Symptoms treated include lack of appetite, fatigue, tired limbs, diarrhea, vomiting, and prolapse.

◆

Tonifies the Lungs. For chronic cough, shortness of breath, copious sputum due to Spleen Chi deficiency.

◆

Nourishes fluids – treating diabetes and thirst.

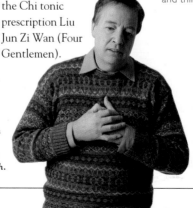

RIGHT *Dang Shen helps to treat symptoms such as shortness of breath.*

Gan Cao

RADIX GLYCYRRHIZAE URALENSIS
Licorice Root

PROPERTIES
Sweet,
Neutral

**CHANNELS
ENTERED**
Lung and
Spleen

Licorice root is sweet and neutral. It is said to enter all 12 channels, and therefore a small quantity is often added to many prescriptions to moderate the effect of Hot and Cold herbs, or to mitigate the harsh properties of other herbs. Its function is often to make a prescription more digestible. It is good for regulating the pulse, but if taken over a long period of time it may cause hypertension (high blood-pressure) or edema (swelling). It is contraindicated in cases of extreme nausea or vomiting.

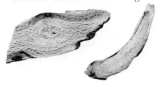

ABOVE *Gan Cao may be
used to regulate the pulse.*

FUNCTIONS AND USES

Tonifies the Spleen and benefits the Chi. Helps tiredness, shortness of breath, and loose stools. For Chi- or Blood-deficient patterns, with irregular pulse or palpitations.

◆

Moistens the Lungs and stops coughing. For any type of coughing or wheezing.

◆

Clears Heat and detoxifies Fire-Poison (toxic sores) — such as carbuncles, sores, or strept throat.

◆

Fried Gan Cao soothes spasms. For painful spasms of the abdomen or legs.

◆

Moderates and harmonizes other herbs.

◆

Antidote for a variety of toxins, taken both internally and applied externally.

Shu Di Huang

RADIX REHMENNIAE GLUTINOSA
Prepared Rehmennia Root

SHU DI HUANG

Shu Di Huang is a very significant herb as it is both a Blood and a Yin tonic. The Kidneys are the basis of both Yin and Jing, the genetic energy which determines a person's constitution. In treating the Jing, Shu Di Huang helps retard the process of aging. It is a very greasy herb and overuse can lead to abdominal distension (bloating) and loose stools, so it must be carefully combined. It is the main ingredient in Liu Wei Di Huang Wan (Six Flavors prescription), the most basic Yin tonic prescription.

PROPERTIES
Sweet, Slightly Warm

CHANNELS ENTERED
Heart, Kidney, Liver

RIGHT ***Shu Di Huang and He Shou Wu act on the Jing.***

FUNCTIONS AND USES

Tonifies the Blood. Symptoms treated include pale complexion, dizziness, palpitations, and menstrual problems.

◆

Nourishes the Yin. For Kidney Yin-deficient patterns, with night sweats, nocturnal emissions, diabetes, and tinnitus (ringing in the ears).

◆

Tonifies Blood and Kidney Jing together. For weak, sore lower back, deafness, weak legs, and premature graying of the hair.

Jing is genetic energy

Jing governs the process of aging

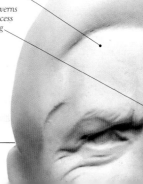

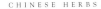

He Shou Wu

HE SHOU WU

RADIX POLYGONUM MULTIFLORUM
Fleeceflower Root (Chinese Cornbind)

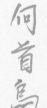

PROPERTIES
Bitter, Sweet,
Astringent,
Slightly Warm

**CHANNELS
ENTERED**
Liver and
Kidney

He Shou Wu is one of the few herbs (together with Shu Di Huang) to help the Jing — therefore it helps prevent the signs of aging when Jing is declining (the name means "black hair"). It lowers blood cholesterol and protects against hardening of the arteries. Like all the moistening herbs, it must be carefully combined to avoid moistening the Spleen too much, leading to diarrhea or phlegm.

FUNCTIONS AND USES

Tonifies the Liver and Kidneys, nourishes the Blood and Jing. Prevents premature graying and loss of hair, spots in front of the eyes (a Liver Blood-deficient sign), weak lower back, and stiffness in the arms and legs.

◆

Firms the Jing and stops leakage. For premature ejaculation, leaking of sperm, and vaginal discharge.

◆

For Fire-Poison — use raw for carbuncles, sores, and goiter.

◆

Moistens the Intestines and unblocks the bowels. Treats constipation, particularly in the elderly.

◆

Expels Wind from the skin by nourishing the Blood. Useful for the treatment of rashes.

◆

Treats malaria — especially when chronic, leading to Chi and Blood deficiency.

Dang Gui

RADIX ANGELICA SINENSIS
Chinese Angelica Root

DANG GUI

PROPERTIES
Sweet, Acrid,
Bitter, Warm

**CHANNELS
ENTERED**
Heart, Liver
and Spleen

Dang Gui is essential in gynecological disorders, as it both tonifies and helps circulation of the Blood. Some herbs used to tonify the Blood are cloying, but Dang Gui is not. It is helpful to add to any prescription for stopping pain, as pain is classified in T.C.M. as caused by either Stagnant Chi or Stagnant Blood. As it is warming, use carefully in Yin-deficient patterns with Heat signs (for example, night sweats).

RIGHT **Dang Gui**
*treats gynecological
problems.*

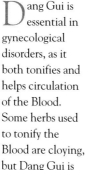

*Improves
menstrual
disorders*

FUNCTIONS AND USES

Tonifies Blood and regulates the menses. For pale complexion, blurred vision, dizziness, palpitations due to deficient Blood. For menstrual disorders associated with Blood deficiency – such as irregular menstruation, amenorrhea (no periods), and dysmenorrhea (period pain).

◆

Invigorates the Blood and disperses Cold – an important herb for stopping pain due to Blood stasis (according to T.C.M.). Treats traumatic injury, abdominal pain, or arthritis.

◆

Moistens the Intestines and unblocks the bowel.

◆

Reduces swelling, expels pus and generates new flesh. Treats sores and abscesses.

Chen Pi

PERICARPIUM CITRUS RETICULATAE
Tangerine Peel

陳
皮

PROPERTIES
Acrid, Bitter,
Warm,
Fragrant

**CHANNELS
ENTERED**
Spleen,
Stomach,
and Lung

Chen Pi is a very important herb as it "awakens the Spleen" to stop it from becoming too Damp, and helps to remove mucus from the chest and diaphragm area. Small doses are added to tonifying prescriptions, in order to make them more digestible. As it is drying (aromatic) and warm, it should be used cautiously in Hot, Dry conditions, such as a dry cough or yellow phlegm.

CHEN PI

FUNCTIONS AND USES

Moves the Chi and strengthens the Spleen. Tackles abdominal bloating, fullness, and lack of appetite.

♦

Dries Dampness and transforms Phlegm – for coughs with a lot of sputum and a feeling of tightness in the chest.

♦

Directs the Chi downward and stops any type of nausea and vomiting.

♦

Helps prevent stagnation – it is put into prescriptions to prevent tonifying, "greasy" herbs causing nausea.

BELOW **Chen Pi
is used to treat
Stagnant Chi.**

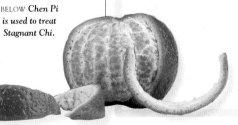

Chuan Xiong

CHUAN XIONG

RADIX LIGUSTICUM WALLICHII
Szechuan Lovage Root

川芎

PROPERTIES
Acrid, Warm

CHANNELS ENTERED
Liver, Gall Bladder and Pericardium

Many gynecological problems are caused by Stagnant Blood, which can be treated by Chuan Xiong. It is also one of the main herbs used for treating headaches (except for migraine caused by rising Liver Yang, as it also moves the Chi to the top of the body), depending on the herbs with which it is combined.

Itchiness is said to be caused by Wind in the skin, and as Chuan Xiong expels wind, it is especially suitable for skin complaints. As it is a warming herb, it must be used with caution in conditions of Deficient Yin with Heat signs. Chuan Xiong is contraindicated for excessive menstrual bleeding, because it moves Blood at a very fast rate.

FUNCTIONS AND USES

Invigorates the Blood and promotes the circulation of Chi. For Stagnant Blood patterns such as dysmenorrhea (period pain), amenorrhea (lack of periods), and difficult labor. Also for pain in the chest and upper abdomen.

✦

Expels Wind and alleviates pain – goes to the top and external parts of the body, and is useful for any headaches, especially those caused by viruses. Also for dizziness, and stiffness due to arthritis. Treats itchy skin caused by Wind.

RIGHT *Painful periods are caused by Stagnant Blood, which can be relieved by Chuan Xiong.*

48

Du Zhong

CORTEX EUCOMMIAE ULMOIDES
Eucommia Bark

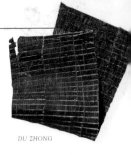

DU ZHONG

Du Zhong tonifies the Liver and Kidneys. As the Liver rules the tendons, and the Kidneys rule the bones, Du Zhong may be used to treat skeletal problems. The Kidneys are put under particular stress during pregnancy, and as Du Zhong is a warming herb, it is used to treat pregnant women who are threatened by miscarriage caused by Cold-deficient Kidney. As a warming herb it is contraindicated in Deficient Yin patterns with Heat signs.

FUNCTIONS AND USES

Tonifies the Liver and Kidneys, strengthens the sinews and bones. For lower back, weak and sore knees, fatigue, leaking of sperm, and frequent urination.

◆

Helps move Chi and Blood. Promotes circulation, especially in the tendons and bones.

◆

Calms the fetus – helps to prevent miscarriage. Good in pregnancy, especially when the woman has lower back pain.

PROPERTIES
Sweet, Slightly Acrid, Warm

CHANNELS ENTERED
Liver and Kidney

LEFT *Pregnancy problems can be ameliorated by taking Du Zhong.*

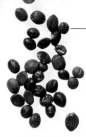

CHINESE HERBAL MEDICINE

Suan Zao Ren

ZIZIPHUS JUJUBA
Sour Date Seed

SUAN ZAO REN

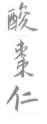

PROPERTIES
Sweet, Sour,
Neutral

**CHANNELS
ENTERED**
Heart, Spleen,
Liver, and
Gall Bladder

Suan Zao Ren is one of the main herbs used for calming the Heart. It is used in combination with other Heart-calming and Blood-tonifying herbs to treat anxiety and emotional problems which have been brought on by Deficient Heart Blood and Yin.

Laboratory tests have proved that Suan Zao Ren has a sedative effect. It must be used cautiously in patients with severe diarrhea. Disturbed Shen (Spirit) also responds to treatment with Suan Zao Ren.

FUNCTIONS AND USES

Nourishes both the Heart and the Liver and calms the Spirit – treats insomnia, palpitations, anxiety, and irritability.

♦

Absorbs sweat – for both spontaneous sweating and night sweats, which are signs of Yin deficiency.

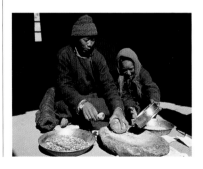

RIGHT **Natural products have been used in the treatment of illness for thousands of years.**

Bai Shao Yao

PAEONIA LACTIFLORA
Peony Root Yao

PROPERTIES
Bitter, Sour,
Cool

**CHANNELS
ENTERED**
Liver and
Spleen

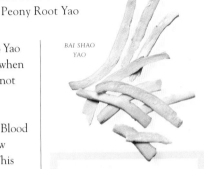

BAI SHAO
YAO

Bai Shao Yao is used when the Liver is not fulfilling its function of making the Blood and Chi flow smoothly. This occurs when the Liver Chi itself has become stuck or "constrained," or when there is disharmony between the Liver and the Spleen, both of which normally have a close relationship in the upper abdomen. Because it is cooling, it tonifies the Blood and Yin – and has a downward action on Heat rising to the head. It anchors the Chi in the Kidneys and therefore, due to the reciprocal relationship between the Liver and the Kidneys, it helps the Kidney Yin to keep the Liver Yang from rising up and causing such symptoms as high blood pressure and headaches.

FUNCTIONS AND USES

Pacifies the Liver and stops pain. Useful for treating flank or chest pain, abdominal cramping, and spasms in the hands and feet. Helps headaches and dizziness due to rising Liver Yang.

◆

Nourishes the Blood. For menstrual dysfunction, vaginal discharge, and uterine bleeding.

◆

Keeps in the Yin and adjusts the fluids. For abnormal or night sweating.

Gui Zhi

RAMULUS CINNAMOMI CASSIAE
Cinnamon Twigs

桂
枝

PROPERTIES
Acrid, Sweet,
and Warm

**CHANNELS
ENTERED**
Lung and
Bladder

Gui Zhi is used mainly for colds and influenza, and commonly in a combination with Bai Shao when there is too much sweating in a cold condition and the patient is becoming weak. It is often added to prescriptions for rheumatic complaints caused by Cold Obstruction causing pain, where it sends warmth through the channels. It is contraindicated in warm diseases.

FUNCTIONS AND USES

Adjusts sweating in externally-caused cold conditions, which helps to eliminate colds.

◆

Warms the meridians and disperses Cold – particularly useful for cold rheumatic complaints, especially in the shoulders.

◆

Moves the Yang and transforms Qi – useful for water retention (edema).

◆

Strengthens the Heart Yang and can be used to treat palpitations.

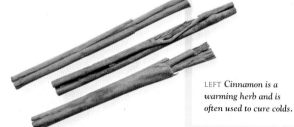

LEFT *Cinnamon is a warming herb and is often used to cure colds.*

Self-help for common ailments

ABOVE **Herbal pharmacies sell a large range of herbs.**

CHINESE HERBAL *treatments are powerful medicines and are best taken under the guidance of an experienced and properly qualified practitioner. Each prescription is carefully balanced for each patient. Taking the wrong medicines in the wrong doses can have unfortunate and even dangerous effects.*

On the whole, Chinese herbs are not designed to be taken singly. There are a number of products sold in health food stores which are made of one herb, such as Wu Wei Zi or Dang Gui. These are fairly safe Chinese herbs, but they are not being used in a traditional way. A qualified Chinese herbalist, will tell you whether a particular patent herbal prescription is suitable, or whether your symptoms are too complicated to be dealt with in such a standardized way.

The dosages on bottles of Chinese patent herbal remedies are often very high. Westerners will usually find it better to start with half the stated dose. If little has changed after five days, then the dosage can be increased by half again.

SELECTING REMEDIES

Chinese remedies are often made up of more than one herb. Therefore, their given names do not always relate to the individual herbal constituents.

Use the following ailments section to work out which remedy is best suited to your complaint. You then need to visit a qualified Chinese herbalist, who will advise you of the correct remedy and its dosage.

ACNE
• Cai Feng Zhen Zhu An Chuang Wan/Margarite Acne Pills. Contains pearl.

ANEMIA
Empty Blood.
• Dang Gui Pian/Angelica Tea. Also tonifies Spleen Chi to help Blood.
• Dang Gui Wan/Angelica Pills. Pure Dang Gui.
• Dang Gui Bu Xue Tang/Tangkuei Decoction. Tonifies the Blood.

ARTERIOSCLEROSIS
Blood stagnation in the Heart and blood vessels.
• Kuan Hsin Su Ho Wan/Cardiovascular Styrax Pills. Also used to prevent heart attacks.

WARNING Do not use during pregnancy.

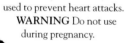

ARTHRITIS AND RHEUMATISM
Caused by invasion of Wind, Cold, or Dampness.
• Du Huo Ji Sheng Wan. For Wind-Damp in the joints, especially lower back and knees.
• Chuan Bi Tang. Especially good for upper back and shoulders.

ASTHMA
Lung Chi or Lung Yin deficiency, possible Kidney Yin or Kidney Yang deficiency, or phlegm.
• Ping Chuan Wan/Calm Asthma Pills. For chronic asthma.
• Qing Qi Hua Ta Tang. For sticky phlegm.

COLDS AND INFLUENZA
• Ganmaoling Pian. For colds and flu, chills, fever, and sore throat.
• Sang Ju Gan Mao Pian. For coughing, runny nose, and congestion.
• Tung Hsuan Li Fei Pian. For headache, fever/chills, and coughs.

CONSTIPATION
Either from Heat, Stagnation of Chi, Deficiency (of Chi, Yang, Blood, or Yin), or Interior Cold.
• Ma Ren Wan. For Heat (dry stools, thirst, dark urine).
• Run Chang Wan. For chronic constipation of any kind.
• Mu Xiang Shun Qi Wan. For Chi stagnation.

COUGHS
Coughs can be Wind-Cold/Heat or Dryness, as well as Damp-Phlegm (white copious phlegm), Phlegm-Heat (yellow sticky phlegm) or, if a deficient-type cough, Lung Chi or Lung Yin deficiency.
• Sang Ju Gan Mao Pian. For dry coughs.
• Ma Xing Zhi Ke Pian. For Wind-Cold or Wind-Heat coughs, acute.
• Chi Kuan Yen Wan. For dry cough with sticky phlegm, or chronic bronchitis with Phlegm-Damp.
• Fritillaria and Loquat Cough Mixture.

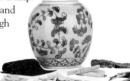

CYSTITIS
Heat or Damp-Heat Painful
Urination syndrome.
• Ba Zheng San/Eight Corrections
Powder.

DEPRESSION
Stagnation of Liver
Chi, which affects
both body and mind.
• Xiao Yao Wan/Free
and Easy Wanderer. Also
treats premenstrual
syndrome.

DIARRHEA
Cold-Damp or Damp-Heat;
Spleen/Stomach deficiency or
Kidney Yang deficiency.
• Huo Xiang Zheng Chi
Wan/Agastache Upright Chi
Powder. For gastric influenza.
• Mu Xiang Shun Qi Wan and Shen
Ling Bai Zhu Wan. Two pills taken
together for alternating diarrhea and
constipation (Liver Chi Stagnation
with Spleen Chi deficiency).
• Liu Jun Zi Pian/Six Gentlemen
Tablet. For loose stools, diarrhea,
indigestion (Spleen Chi deficient).
• Xiang Sha Liu Jun Zi Wan. Same
symptoms with nausea.

DIGESTION, POOR
• Ping Wei Wan/Peaceful Stomach
Tablets. For dyspepsia, abdominal
cramps or bloating, poor appetite,
diarrhea, and nausea.
• Xiang Sha Yang Wei Wan. For
bloating, gurgling, undigested food in
stools, pasty, or erratic stools.

• Shi Chuan Da Bu Wan/Ten
Inclusive Great Tonifying Pills. Take
after illness, weakness, or childbirth.

DYSMENORRHEA
Strong pain – Stagnation of Chi
and Blood, Stagnation of
Cold, Damp-Heat. Weak
pain – Chi and Blood
deficiency, Liver and
Kidney deficiency.
• Xiao Yao Wan/Free and
Easy Wanderer. For
stagnation and pain with
blood clots.
• Wu Ji Bai Feng Wan. For all types
of menstrual disorders.
• Dang Gui Shao Yao Wan. For
Liver and Spleen problems.

EDEMA (WATER RETENTION)
Spleen and Kidney Yang fail to move
and transform water, causing swelling
of the legs or lower abdomen.
• Wu Ling San. Tonifies the Spleen
Yang to resolve edema, particularly of
the lower abdomen.
• Jin Gui Shen Qi Wan. Tonifies the
Kidney Yang to resolve edema,
particularly of the lower legs.

EYE PROBLEMS
Mainly Kidney Yin or Liver Blood
problems, as both these meridians go
to the eyes.
• Qi Ju Di Huang Wan. For blurred
vision, dry, painful eyes, pressure
behind eyes, poor night vision.
• Ming Mu Di Huang Wan. For red
itchy eyes, poor sight, photophobia,
and watery eyes.

FATIGUE

Mainly Chi deficiency or Chi and Blood deficiency.

• Shi Chuan Da Bu Wan. Tonifies Spleen and Heart Chi, Kidney Yang, and nourishes Blood. Fatigue, poor digestion, anxiety, and debility.

• Bu Zhong Yi Qi Wan/Tonify the Centre, Benefit Chi Pill. For Chi deficiency, also for some ME syndromes, as it lightly clears Heat (residual virus).

• Ginseng Royal Jelly Phials. For Spleen and Lung Chi, helps absorption of food.

HAIR LOSS, GRAY HAIR

• Shou Wu Pian. Nourishes Liver Blood, Kidney Chi, and Jing.

HAY FEVER

• Bi Yan Pian/Nose Inflammation Pills. For Wind-Cold or Wind-Heat to the face. Sneezing, itchy eyes, facial congestion and sinus pain, acute and chronic rhinitis, and nasal allergies.

• Yu Ping Feng San/Jade Screen. Helps prevent hay fever, guards against allergies.

• Cang Er Zi Tang/Xanthium Powder. For allergic rhinitis with thicker yellow catarrh or blocked nose.

HEADACHES

Classified by Exterior (sudden, caused by Wind-Cold), or Interior (internal imbalance), and area of headache (meridians affected).

• Chuan Xiong Cha Tiao San. Particularly for sudden headache with a cold or fever.

• Huo Xiang Zheng Qi Wan. From External Dampness (food poisoning, chills) with a dull headache over the forehead.

• Tian Ma Qu Feng Bu Pian. Where Kidney Yin deficiency allows the Liver Yang to rise.

• Tian Ma Gou Teng Yin. Liver Yang Rising headache, on the temples, sides of head and eyebrows.

HYPERTENSION (HIGH BLOOD-PRESSURE)

Mainly deficient Kidney Chi or Yin with hyperactive Liver.

• Fu Fang Du Zhong Pian. Sedates Liver Fire, calms Liver Wind, tonifies Kidney Chi. Characterized by a flushed face, headaches, dizziness, and palpitations.

IMMUNE SYSTEM

• Yu Ping Feng San/Jade Screen. For repeated colds, helps the Wei Chi (defensive energy).

INSOMNIA

Liver or Heart Fire blazing, Phlegm-Heat, Heart and Spleen Blood deficiency, Heart Yin deficiency, Heart and Kidneys not harmonized.

• Gui Pi Wan. Strengthens the Spleen and Heart Chi, Heart Yin and Blood.

• Tian Wang Bu Xin Wan/Heavenly Emperor Tonify the Heart Pill. For

Heart Yin and Blood.
• Suan Zao Ren Tang.
For disturbed mind
(Shen), excessive
dreaming.
• An Mian Pian/
Peaceful Sleep Tablets.
For Heat and congestion in the Liver.

LEUKORRHEA (VAGINAL DISCHARGE)

Damp-Cold (white discharge) or
Damp-Heat (yellow discharge),
involving Damp-Heat in the Kidneys
or Kidney and Spleen Chi deficiency.
• Yu Dai Wan. Classical formula to
heal Damp-Heat in the uterus and
Kidney.
• Zhi Bai Ba Wei Wan. Kidney Yin
deficient leukorrhea, with hot
flushes, night sweating, restless sleep.
• Bu Zhong Yi Qi Wan. For Spleen
Chi deficiency with Damp, with
tiredness, shortness of breath, loose
stools.

LOWER BACKACHE

• Yao Tong Pian. For deficiency of
Kidney Yang (back pain in the
kidney area).

MALE SEXUAL PROBLEMS

• Jin Suo Gu Jing Wan/Golden Lock
Tea. Tonifies Kidney Yang. For
seminal discharge and premature
ejaculation.

MENOPAUSE

• Liu Wei Di Huang Wan/Six Flavor
Rehmennia Pill. Tonifies the Kidney
Yin, which declines in old age.

NAUSEA AND VOMITING

Also see Digestion.
• Er Chen Wan. Dissolves Phlegm,
resolves Spleen Damp and Harmonizes
the Centre (digestive organs).

PAIN, DIGESTIVE

• Mu Xiang Shun Qi Wan. For dull
epigastric pain, worse with pressure,
belching, sour regurgitation, foul
breath, vomiting of undigested food.
• Shu Gan Wan. For pain and
distention clearly related to the
emotional state, feeling of pressure in
the chest, slight breathlessness,
belching.
• Bao He Wan. For abdominal pain,
worse with pressure and after eating,
feeling of fullness in the stomach,
diarrhea which relieves the pain, or
constipation.

PHLEGM

Phlegm in the Lungs, throat, and
nasal passages.
• Qing Qi Hua Ta Tang/Clean
Air Tea/Pinellia Expectorant
Pills. For bronchial or sinus
congestion, asthma.
• Zhi Sou Ding Chuan Wan.
For asthma with cough and
sticky phlegm.

PREMENSTRUAL SYNDROME (PMS)

Mainly due to Liver Chi
stagnation.
• Xiao Yao Wan/ Free and Easy
Wanderer. For breast tenderness,
moodiness, and clumsiness.
• Yue Ju Wan. Helps depression.

• Chai Hu Su Gan Tang. Particularly for pain in the breasts, and swelling.

PROLAPSE
• Bu Zhong Yi Qi Wan. For prolapse of uterus, rectum, and colon, due to deficiency of Chi and Yang. Also for hemorrhoids, varicose veins, and hernia. Useful for uterine bleeding, habitual miscarriage, and chronic diarrhea.

SINUSITIS
• Bi Yan Pian. Very good for sinusitis, especially with sticky yellow nasal discharge, hard to get out.
• Cang Er Zi San. For lots of green nasal discharge, headache, and pain.
• Xin Yi San. For lots of clear or white nasal discharge, nasal congestion and pain.

SORE THROAT
• Yin Qiao Jie Du Pian. Flu symptoms, swollen lymph nodes, and headaches.
• Sang Ju Gan Mao Pian or Sang Ju Yin Pian. For cold symptoms.
• Liu Wei Di Huang Wan. For Kidney Yin-deficient sore throat, and chronic dry sore throat, with hot palms and soles, and night sweats.

TINNITUS
Can be divided into excess conditions (Rising of Liver and Gall Bladder Fire, Phlegm-Fire) and Kidney or Jing Deficiency leading to weak Liver Yang rising.
• Long Dan Xie Gan Wan. For excess conditions; sudden onset, loud sound, related to emotional strain, irritability, possibly with red eyes, thirst, and constipation.
• Er Ming Zuo Ci Wan/Tso-Tzu Otic Pills. For Kidney Yin deficiency with Liver Fire rising; gradual onset, low sound, slight dizziness, poor memory, blurred vision, sore back and knees, and low sexual desire.

TONSILLITIS
• Liu Shen Wan/Six Spirits Pill. Not for sore throat in the early stages of a Wind attack, but for real tonsillitis. For strept infection, you may need to combine it with another prescription. **WARNING** Contains animal products. Prohibited in pregnancy.

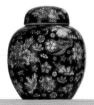

Further reading

Williams, Tom, THE COMPLETE ILLUSTRATED GUIDE TO CHINESE MEDICINE (Element Books, 1996)

Kaptchuk, Ted J., THE WEB THAT HAS NO WEAVER (Congdon and Weed, 1983)

Bensley, D. and Gamble, A., CHINESE HERBAL MEDICINE MATERIA MEDICA (Eastland Press, 1993)

Fratkin, Jake, CHINESE HERBAL PATENT REMEDIES, A PRACTICAL GUIDE (Institute for Traditional Medicine, Portland, Oregon, 1986)

Hyatt, Richard, CHINESE HERBAL MEDICINE, ANCIENT ART AND MODERN SCIENCE (Wildwood House Limited, 1978)

Useful addresses

U.K.
The Register of Chinese Herbal Medicine (RCHM)
PO Box 400
Wembley
Middlesex
HA9 9NZ
Tel: 0181 904 1357

British Acupuncture Council (BAC)
Park House
206-208 Latimer Road
London
W10 6RE
Tel: 0181 964 0222

AUSTRALIA
Australian Natural Therapist Association
PO Box 308
Melrose Park 5039
Tel: +61 8 297 9533

U.S.A.
American Association of Oriental Medicine (AAOM)
433 Front Street
Catasauqua
PA 18032
Tel: +1 610 2661433

National Accreditation Commission for Schools and Colleges of Acupuncture and Oriental Medicine (NACSCAOM)
1010 Wayne Avenue
Suite 1270
Silver Springs
MD 20910
Tel: +1 301 6089680

American Oriental Bodywork Association
50 Maple Place
Manhasset
NY 19030